PRAISE FOR ONEDERLAND

"A person's creative process is inevitably shaped by that person's experiences. I am moved by Jamie's sharing of her thoughts in these poems and impressed with her ability to do so eloquently and provocatively. Jamie's poetry is lovely and deals with a variety of subjects. Type 1 diabetes certainly doesn't define Jamie, but it is undeniably a part of her (until we succeed in curing it!). I am grateful that she helps us all better understand her life, and by extension the lives of others."

—**Derek Rapp**, Former president & CEO of JDRF

"*Onederland* is an impressive coming-of-age effort by Jamie Kurtzig. Her debut collection of poetry cleverly reframes Type 1 diabetes as a character in what is a beautifully crafted exploration of growing up, both with chronic illness and in today's world generally. Jamie's work is an exciting display of talent from the next generation of writers."

—**Thom Scher**, CEO of Beyond Type 1

"In *Onederland: My Childhood with Type 1 Diabetes,* young poet Jamie Kurtzig opens her heart and shares her struggle with the highs and lows of a chronic illness that she has faced since age one. The work shines with her bright, brave perspective."

> —**Linda Watanabe McFerrin**,
> Author of *Namako, The Hand of Buddha*, and
> *Navigating the Divide*

"Vibrant and alive, this work is also amazingly delicate and fragile; Jamie has refined each line to the most precise reflection of her intricate, sensitive mind. In poems full of the triumphs and the tests of being a teenager, she brings us right to the heart of human feeling, human hope, and human resilience. It's a book that inspires courage, smiles, and compassion—written by someone who clearly has all of them in abundance to share."

> —**Cole Swenson**, Author of *On Walking On*

"Any poet who uses 'interstitial fluid' in one of her rhymes is a woman after my heart - or, in this case, a teenager after my heart. Jamie Kurtzig brings uncommon maturity to her writing, demonstrating that youth can be its own inspiration. Jamie writes eloquently, and thoughtfully, about the search for a cure for type 1 diabetes. May she live long enough to see her wish fulfilled."

—**James S. Hirsch**, Author of *Cheating Destiny*

ONEDERLAND

MY CHILDHOOD WITH TYPE 1 DIABETES

ONEDERLAND

MY CHILDHOOD WITH TYPE 1 DIABETES

JAMIE KURTZIG

MAKEHISTORYPRESS

❧

I never expected to be a poet. As I was cleaning out my childhood treasures, I discovered that I had written many poems (you can see my original poems on the first few pages). After giving a small packet of poems to my grandmas as holiday gifts, I decided to continue telling my life story through poetry. At that moment, the idea of *Onederland* was born.

My poetry book, *Onederland*, is a collection of 100 poems that I wrote from kindergarten to high school. The poems cover topics ranging from Type 1 diabetes to sunsets to worn-out shoes. By purchasing a copy and looking at the world through my eyes, you will be supporting Type 1 diabetes non-profits and their groundbreaking work toward finding a cure and improving the lives of millions of children and people, like me, who live with Type 1 diabetes. I have been living with Type 1 diabetes since I was one year old, and it is my dream to be a part of finding the cure.

—Jamie Kurtzig

ISBN-978-1-7331819-1-4

First Edition/first Printing
Printed in the United States of America

This book is dedicated to
all living with Type 1 diabetes,
all who live in Oneder,
all who are writing in between the Once-Upon-a-Time
and the Happily-Ever-After,
Mom, who teaches me to make lemonade out of lemons
and who loves me enough for anything,
Dad, who reminds me to always keep trying (Imua!),
Kelly, who teaches me to spread positive energy like
spreading frosting on a cake,
Kai, who teaches me to find the good in everyone
("I love you, stranger!"),
Mimi, who loves me to the moon and back infinity and
beyond times, and
Glamma, for paving the way.

Author's Note

I decided to call my poetry book *Onederland* because I have had Type 1 diabetes since I was 1 year old, I want my blood sugar numbers to stay in the **100s** (my family and I have gotten in the habit of calling the **100s** "**Onederland**"), and I have **100** poems in my book.

Type 1 diabetes is a lifelong and 24/7 condition without a cure. Because I have Type 1 diabetes, my pancreas doesn't work as well as it should. The pancreas is an organ inside the body that produces insulin, a hormone that controls blood sugar. My pancreas doesn't make insulin. I did nothing to get this condition. Type 1 diabetes is an autoimmune disease with genetic predispositions (no one in my family has Type 1 diabetes, but there is a history of other autoimmune diseases in my family) and an environmental trigger (unknown as of now).

This is what it is like to live with Type 1 diabetes: Imagine getting a needle poked into your body where your insulin must be delivered. Imagine having another needle in your arm to track your blood sugar levels. Imagine needing to sit out every time your blood sugar goes low to regain your thinking and yourself. This is what Type 1 diabetes means for me. However, the scariest part is how I could die from this condition like I almost did after an accidental insulin overdose. These are some reasons why one of my main life goals is to help find a cure for Type 1 diabetes and why I am donating the money raised from this book to nonprofits that support Type 1 diabetes research and cures.

Thank you so much for reading my book!

Swshh
Swshh

God is
watering the
Earth to make
people happy
Swshh, swshh
Rain
by
Jamie

"Rain" my very first poem

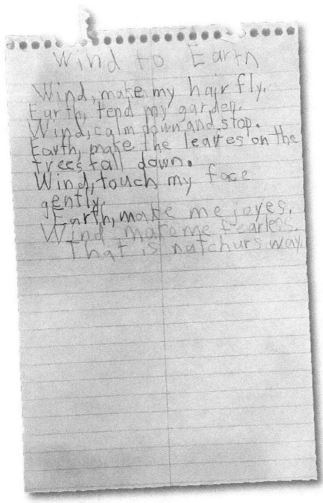

"Wind to Earth", a handwritten poem from second grade

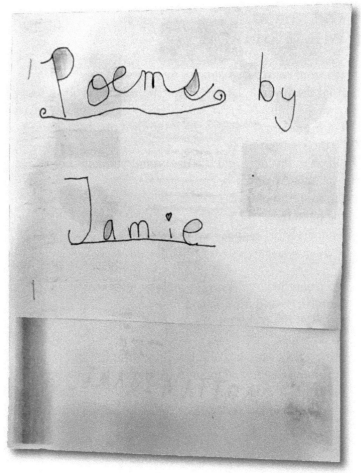

My poetry packet given to my grandmas
was the inspiration for my *Onederland* book.

WHERE I'M FROM

I'm from continuous glucose monitors,
from the Juvenile Diabetes Research Foundation
    and Ifshin.
I'm from the wildness of the overgrown plants hiding
    their secrets away.
(Blazing, dry, deer and lizards running through the
    parched plants.)
I'm from the plumeria tree and
the palm tree
I remember climbing,
inching up, searching for their blossoms.

I'm from the party throwers and the rational ones,
from Brody and Mulholland.
I'm from the techies and
the sporties,
from try-your-hardest and live-life-to-the-fullest.
I'm from science and modern technology:
the belief in evolution
that is shaping us today.

I'm from between Parker and Maple,
challah, charoset, and spuds,
from the stories my Grandma Brody told while acting
    as a boy,
to the eye my great-grandfather lost while fighting fires,
and the lesson Grandma Gigi taught me: "Life is short
    but sweet."

Underneath my books lie
the pieces of my own history:
the very photographs, old drawings, and relics
that my drop of water condensed from.
I'm from the sea of memories—
the sea that flows as one, goes as one,
yet each drop makes the ocean bigger and
    more beautiful.

SPARRING TOURNAMENT

I put my headgear on and my mouthpiece in.
I step into the arena to shake hands with my opponent.
She is a little taller than I am and wears
her hair in a braid sprouting from her headgear.

A coach tells me:
"Just a last-minute
rule change.
There will be
headshots in this fight."

Headshots? I have practiced headshots a
few times.
No problem, I think.
No problem at all.

The referee orders:
"*Chung. Hung.*" Blue. Red.
He points to our starting spots
with straight arms, looking straight forward.

"*Si Jahk!*" Begin.

I bounce on my toes, and
we move in a circle for what seems like forever.
Boom! She rushes at me and does an
inside crescent kick before I can reach my hands
   up to block.
I see my mom jump to her feet.

❧

I shake it off.
I keep bouncing on my toes, and
I get a close enough distance so that I can do
a spinning back hook kick.
I know these spinning kicks earn extra points.

I spin around, but then she
kicks me with her own sliding hook kick.

It's right in the head.
No, that time it was in my face.

She rushes at me again, and I
hear my coach yell: "Keep your arms up!"
I raise my arms up, but she spins into a
360° jumping roundhouse kick
and then an outside crescent kick to my head.
It is all I can do to push her away with an axe kick.

I look at the scoreboard: 10-1.
I remember headshots earn extra points.
30 seconds have passed. I have
1 minute and 30 seconds left.

Bam! Another sliding hook kick and then
a back hook kick that hits hard and
brushes across my face.
My eyes are like fire, and it feels like
fire trucks spray them with salty water.

A tear drops down on the floor.

I get in really close to her, trying to
execute my jump-away roundhouse kick,
but my body feels like I weigh 300 pounds. My
jump-away roundhouse kick looks more like a
stumble-away-get-my-leg-up kick.

She comes after me with a sequence of 3 different kicks:
one at my face, one on my *hogu*, and another to my face.
She drives me to the outskirts of the arena, and I
step out.

"Kyong-go!" Warning before a point deduction.

Like the score could be any more uneven.
"Kae sok!" Continue.
She advances toward me.

My face feels white and red at the same time.
Is my nose bleeding?
My feet do not bounce anymore.

She kicks and kicks. I hunch over
and hope she doesn't kick my head again.
Strong kick to the head. I careen over.

My mom rushes over: "Sweetie, do you want to stop
the fight?"
I try to talk, but it takes a while for me to regain my
breath.
"Mom, I only have one minute left. How bad can
one minute be?"
"Gamjeom!" Full point deduction.
I get up.
She kicks me.

CAN'T

You're just a
girl.
You'll
never be a
doctor or a scientist.
You can't be good at
math.

You're just a
kid.
You can't have a job
or do anything valuable.
You're just too young and
inexperienced.

You have celiac disease.
You can't eat cake or be
a baker or pastry chef.
It's just that all this
food has gluten.

Not true.

CELIAC DISEASE

No normal bread
or soy sauce.
No normal pasta or pizza
or muffins or cereal.

"No cross contamination."
"No thank you. I'll pass."
"Please be careful."

Name

showing who i am
belongs to me

Student

Never stop learning—
ever.
No one knows everything.

Doctor

stitching the great world
determined hands move gently

HIGH BLOOD SUGAR

feel thirsty
water tastes sugary

feel dizzy
need to sit down

not eating
lying down, lacking energy

alarms beeping
people staring

bolusing
how much insulin should i give?

looks like texting
phone taken away

throw up

CLOCK

ticking, ticking on
through the day and through the night
forever counting

hands always moving
ticking to infinity
ticking, ticking on

COURAGE

Courage is purple.
It tastes like plums.
It smells like hot oatmeal with syrup,
reminds me of the Statue of Liberty.
It sounds like a hummingbird flapping its wings.
Courage makes me feel brave.

QUARTET

"Here's what I'm thinking,"
says my violin teacher.
"This will be a stretch,
but I want to put you
in this quartet."

He shows it to me,
and I swallow a gasp.
He'd really put me with them
and almost guarantee a crash?

But, I hear myself saying,
"Okay, this sounds great. I will
practice a lot."

"Yes, you'll have to,"
he says.
I know that.

After my lesson,
I think some more
and then I decide
how to proceed.

It's good to challenge myself,
and this is a time for growth.
I will learn for next time,
and I bet I won't crash after
practicing so much.

So, I decided to stay in the advanced quartet.
I'm ready.

AUDITION

I walk in with my violin and
its shiny E-string tuner.
Bizet's Symphonie en Ut, second movement.
I hand my conductor my evaluation sheet
with a shaky hand and a
forced smile.

I place the tip of my bow on the string.
Piano. Espressivo.
I begin my *crescendo* and first shift.

I think back to my practices.

I did practice, and I
practiced every day
so that I could get a better seat.
When I finished my homework
at eleven at night, I still practiced.
I want a better seat.

I am tired of sitting in the back.
I am fourth chair, but everyone moves
in front of me, so
I sit in the back row
by myself
with the back of my chair touching
the exit door.

✍

I move on to the faster part,
where I play *spiccato*.

No missed notes. No stroke malfunctions. No crashes.
Just me playing my violin.

It is done. I have finished my audition,
but how did I do?

Two weeks later, I see an email.
The note reads, "I know some of you may be
disappointed with your seating audition results."
I skip the rest and open the document.

I look for my name,
but not for long.
"Jamie Kurtzig" is under "first violin"—
and "first chair."

MUSIC

I don't just want to play notes
on a page.

I want to play *crescendos*
and *decrescendos*,

legato and *spiccato*,
espressivo and *allegro*.

Yes, I want to play it all

because music is so much more
than notes on a page.

HOW LONG IS A MOMENT?

How long is a moment?
Does it last a second,
the duration of a blink,
every time I smile?

How long is a moment?
Does it last a nanosecond,
the length of every breath,
each time I learn something?

How long is a moment?
Does it last a minute,
the time between each step,
every time I do an act of kindness?

How long is a moment?

ORGANIZATION

perfection
tidy and neat
like out of a
picture book

made bed,
color-coded clothes,
clear desk,
filed papers

simple

☙

Taekwondo

learning to be calm and relaxed—
even in the midst of chaos

mastering the art of patience
with others and one's self

sharp and graceful movement
flowing together in harmony

balancing both
yin and yang

defending and standing up for people
who cannot do it themselves

facing adversity with
balance and grace

FREE VERSE

no rules
no limitations
nothing you can't do

just keep going
keep thinking
write it down

you can write about soaring in an airplane
or getting the flu,
something found in everyday life
or about something extraordinary that hasn't happened twice

free verse is where you have the liberty
to write a poem of your choice
take that abstract thought
and put it into reality
that is free verse poetry

WATER

drop
water
on my tongue
tastes refreshing
cleansing my body of hurt
helping me keep on keeping on
another drop is coming from the sky
i'm catching it on my tongue this time
it helps me to move on to the present
refreshing my senses, renewing me
everything is going to be okay
there's no need to worry
i'm good now

PI

an endless sea—
a sea of digits

they swim
in and out
of minds

constantly more
constantly flowing

we will never find an end

THINK

What do I need to multiply by
$x + yi$
to produce the real number
$T + 0i$?

Identify poetic devices in the
Twelfth Night quote:
"...like a worm i' th' bud, feed on her damask cheek."

What is the
significance of the
1917 Bolshevik Revolution?

Why does racism exist?

What is the
Endosymbiosis Theory for how
chloroplasts and mitochondria
exist in prokaryotes?

En una cláusula adverbial,
como puedo conjugar "decírselo"
si "a pesar de que" es antes del verbo?

Is this chord a tritone,
a diminished seventh,
or a third?

CRACKING KNUCKLES

Crack! I twist my finger.
Pop! Then I pull on it.
Snap! Next finger.

"Relax your hands,"
my mom commands.

She still hears
all the cracking
and popping
and snapping.

"Why would you do that?"
she asks.

I circle my neck now.
Crack!
Pop!
Snap!

It helps me
get my nerves out.

Long silence.

I twirl my wrists.
Crack!
Pop!
Snap!

She puts her hand
over my hands.
"Stop."

PROCRASTINATION

Everything is fine.
I'll just watch a movie now
and do it later.

"It will be okay,"
I say after the movie.
"I have tomorrow."

"I'll take a walk now.
I'll do it this afternoon,"
I say to myself.

It's due in an hour,
I realize after walking.
What am I to do?

BROKEN

shattered
into
millions
of pieces

will never
be the
same
again

cannot
be fixed

STRESS

5 pounds
10 pounds
2 pounds
3 pounds
5 pounds
I accept the weights.
It's fun.

25 pounds
I'm not too
bad at this.

I take more—
15 pounds
7 pounds
8 pounds
Wow, that was fast.
55 pounds now.

My legs start to quake.
I feel a drop of sweat
form on my forehead.
I can't wipe it off—
my hands are full.

20 pounds
I teeter-totter back and forth.
Spectators laugh.
I won't quit in front of them.

15 pounds
My arms feel like lead.

10 pounds
I close my eyes.
Deep breaths through the pain.

100 pounds now
It's like a show—
how much can I take?

I am like the Leaning
Tower of Pisa.
When
will I fall?

LOW BLOOD SUGAR

hungry
choking as many glucose tabs
down as i can

they taste like sawdust and tart combined

legs won't work
just enough energy
to eat glucose tabs

can you get me a glass of water?

shaky hands
pale face
like the glucose tabs i eat

i drink some juice, too

annoying alarm
"shhh!"
"why are you eating in class?"

sorry, didn't mean to distract you

slow blinks
deep breaths
sweating

wait, what did you say?

"are you good?"
you know what,
can you just stop?

and, yes, everything is perfectly fine

SADNESS

Sadness is grey.
It tastes like
soggy bread.

It smells like photos of
my great-grandparents who have passed on,
and reminds me of rain

filling up my boots.
It sounds like
people crying, quietly

with their heads in their hands.
Sadness makes me feel like
my problems are

small and insignificant.

TRASHCAN

a bin showered with hate—
anger and frustration
thrive,

a bin where there is no rebirth,
only death

a bin where important
items
are soon forgotten,
an enormous bin threatening
to shroud
the world

a bin that reeks
from the stench
of broken dreams

SILENCE

a place of no opinion
too scared to speak out
too scared to stand up
too scared of having a voice

sometimes it is harder to say the first word
than all of the ones following it

꧁

FAMILY

strong like a boulder—
every day, welcoming me to
climb it

or simply sit on it
to watch the
clouds move above me

yet it is fun like a puddle—
I can run through it
in my rainboots

and jump up high
to see the waves and ripples
I can make

once a member steps into
my circle of hope,
they are always a part of me

FIRST DAY OF HIGH SCHOOL

pick out the perfect outfit
comb your hair
brush your teeth for five minutes

"do i look okay?"

get in the car
don't be late
you'll be fine
make friends
have fun

it's not that easy

arriving
fake smile on top of nervousness
"hi! i'm jamie!"
name games
cheesy bonding activities
"what's your name again?"

lunch line.
"can i sit with you?"
"of course!"

COLD

I flee out the front door,
and I run to catch the bus,
but I feel something's off.

I got my backpack, my textbook,
my book, so
what could I be forgetting?

I shiver and rub my arms,
then remember—

my jacket.

Fashion

There once was a girl coming to school
that wanted to pick out clothes that looked cool.
She tried on eight dresses and six shoes,
but she forgot it was cold like igloos.
Next year she'll do the "check-the-weather" rule.

BEAUTY

look past appearance
allure is seen by true friends
hearts contain beauty

BOOK

a picture—
a picture without paint
can make you laugh
or cry

a puzzle,
but it has no pieces

a flow of emotions
and a wonderful page-turner

Rainy Day

warm, fuzzy blankets
sitting by the fireplace
reading books on the couch
chili and cornbread

looking through windows,
watching rain fall

drip drop
pitter patter
drip drop

GLASSES

When you see a glass of water,
it is half full
and erupts with
fireworks,
adventure,
and love.

When I see a glass of water,
it is half empty
and only looks like
a normal glass.

I say that it is a different glass.
No, you tell me,
it is something else.
Then,
my eyes open to
imagination.

PEN

pick it up
yes
for with this tool
the world
will be changed
forever

IMAGINATION

a freedom for one
a prison for another

POEMS

creativity
everything out on paper
forever-lasting

Butterfly's Wingbeat

small, but effective
makes the world a better place
peacefully, smoothly

☙

SUMMER DAY

I open my curtains,
and then I open the door.

I walk outside—
what a delightful day!

ENERGY

green grass
blowing bubbles:
chasing them and
giggling when i pop them

bright blue sky
shining sun
silly songs
bursting into laughter

merry go round
watermelon smiles
playing tag
beautiful summer day

SURPRISE

like waking up
to the smell of french toast
and maple syrup

like a friend texting me,
"when do you want
to hang out?"

like seeing the last
gluten-free chocolate chip
cookie waiting for me

like looking out
the kitchen window
just in time for sunset

like finding the perfect
shell on the beach
to add to my collection

like when i get to choose
the tv show
we watch on friday nights

like spotting a shiny
penny on monday's
gray sidewalks

GOLD

Which one?
A fortune of gold?
Or a heart of gold?
Which should I choose?

I see a banquet of filet mignon
and lobster, too.

Servants escort me to
my own limousine,
and I put on my 24-karat gold ring
encrusted with diamonds.

or...

I hold the door open,
and I high-five
a young boy.

I tell a classmate how amazing
she is at chess.
She beams back, and she
shares a cookie with a friend.

I invite the new kid
to hang out with me
this afternoon.
She tells our teacher
she loves learning about biology.

And one day,
someone gives me
flowers.

CHOCOLATE

texture of perfection
i take a bite
bliss washes over me
the rich creamy flavor
melts in my mouth

∽

BLUE

a vast sea
of tranquility
bliss and calmness all around
laughter if it was a sound

∾

SNIFFER

He's an
orange and purple
stuffed dog.

He's slept on my bed
the past 13 years,
but now,
should I move him
to a shelf in my closet?

PEN PALS A WORLD APART

A person like me is
small compared to the world.
How can I help unite it
if I am just one kid?

I write a little letter in Spanish
with pictures of
my family
to a preschooler who loves to sing.

Mail from my pen pal
arrives on my front porch.
There is a drawing of a butterfly
and a letter of thanks I read in Spanish.

I ignore the translated English part.
Why am I so lucky
to have a friend
this incredible?

BIRTHDAY PRESENTS

I wanted a thoroughbred horse
that could run really quickly
when I was seven.

I did not get a horse.

I wanted a lock for my door
to keep my siblings out
when I was eight.

I did not get a lock.

I wanted more recess time
to play with my friends
when I was nine.

I did not get more recess time.

I wanted to go out of the country
to China for the first time
when I was ten.

I did not go to China.

I wanted to be the fastest runner
in cross country and track
when I was eleven.

❧

I did not win first place.

I wanted to grow
to at least five feet
when I was twelve.

I did not grow taller.

I wanted to get into every high school
I applied to
when I was thirteen.

I did not get into every high school.

I wanted love
from my friends and family
when I was fourteen.

I got love.

¿POR QUÉ?

Quiero aprender español.
Quiero comunicarme con mucha gente,
y no quiero que una
barrera del idioma me detenga
Viajé a Costa Rica, Panamá, y México,
pero no podía entender sus acentos
y lo rápido que hablaban.
¿Cómo puedo entenderlos?
En clase de español,
mi maestra me dijo que
necesito mejorar mi pronunciación porque
dije PA-na-ma y no Pa-na-MÁ.
Un día,
quiero hablar con los lugareños
en español sin
ninguna vacilación.
¿Por qué?
Porque hay tantas
personas extraordinarias que quiero conocer
que hablan idiomas además de
inglés.

∽

WHY? (English Translation)

I want to learn Spanish.
I want to communicate with many people,
and I do not want a language barrier to stop me.
I traveled to Costa Rica, Panama, and Mexico,
but I couldn't understand their accents
and how quickly they spoke.
How can I understand them?
In Spanish class,
my teacher told me that
I need to improve my pronunciation because
I said PA-na-ma and not Pa-na-MA.
One day,
I want to talk with the locals
in Spanish without
any hesitation.
Why?
Because there are so many
extraordinary people I want to meet
who speak languages besides
English.

UKRAINE

I see a blue and yellow flag.
They say it represents
the sky and the
fields below.

But, the flag is more than that.

It's blue for tears shed
from war and signs saying
"Free all Ukrainian
political prisoners."

It's yellow for gold people standing still
and taking pictures with
me for money.

It's blue for the rain
pouring down
while Ukrainian kids pass the
soccer ball to my brother,
and he passes back.

It's yellow for the shiny
trumpet playing
patriotic songs each day from
a balcony.

It's blue for the shirt I wore while a
little girl played beautiful
pieces on the violin.
Her case was open for money.

It's yellow for the flaming coffee desserts
we enjoyed underground.

It's blue for the old woman's scarf
while she sat on the
side of the gravel road
in her rocking chair
next to a small shack
that looked like it was falling down.

It's blue for OST badges
and yellow for the Star of David
that Ukrainians and Ukrainian Jews
had to wear during the time when
synagogues turned into theatres.

Ukraine is like the
smooth statue of a stone bull
with a girl sitting on its horns.

MAYBE

I used to think maybe meant yes—
back when I was little.
There would be problems,
but everything would turn out fine.
All stories used to end with a happily-ever-after.

I used to think maybe meant no—
some things could never be,
no matter how much I tried.
Continuing to haunt me,
they would always be like that.
Only fairy tales used to be a happily-ever-after.

Now, maybe means maybe—
not yes, not no,
just maybe.
This story will maybe have a happily-ever-after.
Just maybe.

BAD GRADE

They call me a
perfectionist, a
worry-wart, a
stressed-out student.

They imitate me
in high-pitched voices:
"Oh no! I got an 88% on the test.
It's the end of the world!"

But to me, it really does matter.

〰

Wind to Earth

Wind, make my hair fly.
Earth, tend my garden.

Wind, calm down and stop.
Earth, make the leaves on the trees fall down.

Wind, touch my face gently.
Earth, make me joyous.

Wind, make me fearless.

That is nature's way.

BLACK SAND BEACH

boogie board
goggles
towel

That's all that's on this beach.

It's my very own paradise
with colorful coral,
a jagged lava rock
poking
just out of the water,
swaying palm trees.

I smile,
run to the water—
free like a *humu humu* fish.

ALOHA'S SYMPHONY

I hear a symphony:
crashing waves are cellos, playing *tremolo* after *tremolo*;
peaceful winds, blowing through palm trees, are flutes,
    pianissimo, yet still there;
playful dolphins' laughter are trumpets, playing *allegro;*
a humpback whale's song (catching sun's rays on blue
    skin)
is the solo violinist, vivaciously vibrating every *cantante*
    note.

I see figures on our black sand beach sometimes:
they drink strawberry lilikoi smoothies in flip flops with
    sandy toes,
swoop into cerulean blue crests of waves,
shaka to their friends,
smiling brighter than daylight's reflection on the ocean.

If I were one of them,
I would drive in my faded, yellow bug car (surfboard
    atop)
to the hidden black sand beach every day,
and I would pass a plumeria lei to everyone I saw.

A small noise like *pizzicato*
turns my head to see these gigantic eyes
springing from an egg as if she just popped a balloon.
She has a green shell like mine,
weak flippers cannot yet support the enormous weight
    of those irises.
I wave my own flipper toward the setting sun, and to-
    gether,
we watch him lay his head on the pillow of the horizon.

I glide with her as she learns to take her first steps,
inching toward the ocean, slowly, steadily.
She takes a deep breath before ducking
her head under the threshold between air and water:
the symphony plays on.

SHOOTING STAR

I wish for treasure:
the treasures of kindness, love.
I don't long for gold.

Look, a shooting star!
Please help me find this treasure;
I hope you hear, star.

EYELASHES

I close my eyes
and make a wish.

I blow softly and
hope it travels far.

FLOATING WISH LANTERN

I see the lanterns.
They glow and float in the sky.
What will my wish be?

❧

LUNAR NEW YEAR

a glistening ball of light
rises and falls
in a rhythmic pattern
watches
a celebration
that makes
magic
and myths
come
to
life

HAPPINESS

Happiness is yellow.
It tastes like lilikoi pudding.
It smells like plumerias
and reminds me of Hawaiian sunsets at the beach.
It sounds like people laughing.
Happiness makes me feel cheerful.

HAIKU

This is a haiku.
I hope you enjoy reading.
It is just for you!

Five, seven, and five:
composed out of syllables—
fun to read and write.

Very intriguing,
a beautiful form of art—
complex poetry.

Many are funny,
others can be dramatic,
serious ones, too.

Haikus are funny,
but this one is not funny.
Oh well, I tried hard.

Flying

I am leaping
in my garden,
flowers blossoming
at my feet.
I am going as quickly
as it takes
a butterfly
to
take flight.

I pretend
to fly,
coast, and
soar
like a real
bird.

MOON

Tonight, we are up:
when I am doing homework
way past my bedtime;

when I lie in bed
not dreaming, but worrying,
tossing, and turning;

when I turn off the lights,
and no one can say "goodnight"
since they are asleep.

So, tonight, it's just us:
the glittering moon and me.

A FEELING

As I reach out to touch the heart that has touched me,
an immense feeling shrouds me.

A feeling stronger than a lion,
but it will not harm me.

A feeling more powerful than hate,
but it does not hate me.

A feeling more compassionate than a dove,
but it will not fly away.

A feeling more stunning than the sound of the sea,
but it never breaks.

FLOWER

all unique
all an earth's piece
blossoms into beauty
a burst of color
this wonderful living thing

WISHING FOR TYPE 1 DIABETES

She says,
"You are so lucky
you have Type
1 diabetes."

"Wait,
did I mishear you?
Did you say you
wish you had
Type 1 diabetes?"

"Yes.
You get so much
attention,
and you get to eat
those sugary things."

"First of all,
those glucose tabs
are medical treatments,
and they taste
terrible.

⌒

When I have low blood sugars
because of my Type 1 diabetes,
I feel out of energy,
unable to think,
and unable to be myself.

High blood sugars
because of Type 1 diabetes
make me
throw up
and feel terrible.

Before insulin shots,
people died
from Type 1 diabetes.

You should be the one
feeling lucky."

SEASONS

In fall,
the sunflowers stand tall.
I stomp in the leaves:
no more pet peeves.

Winter can freeze:
I stand in the cold wind with ease.
I hope that tomorrow
I can look out my window and see snow!

In spring,
all the flowers sing.
Flowers abloom,
you won't find me in my room!

Summer,
the opposite of a bummer:
the perfect time to get sprayed by a hose.
Everything is sweaty, even my toes.

SUMMER

How long will it be until summer?
Or until I drink water with cucumber?
I'm really pretty tired,
but summer makes me inspired.
Oh, when can I be sunlight's newcomer?

JUMP

encouragement

"Do it!"
"Just go!"
"Everything will be fine!"
"Make us proud!"
"Make yourself proud!"

hesitation

No.
Hold on.
Will everything be fine?
I can't do it.
I'm just not strong enough.

trust

Yes.
This is going to be fun.
I will be fine.
Of course I can do it.
I will be so proud of myself.

jump

and fly

THE TASTE OF VICTORY

now is the time;
practicing for this moment,
envisioning success

but now, after
dreaming for this moment,
it's here

the hours of effort kick in,
so close to dreams coming true

it's a blur;
i'm finished

the taste is overwhelming:
the taste of victory, sweet

FENCING

En garde,
ready,
fence!

I advance:
my foil in my right hand,
my left hand by
my side.

I advance.
They advance.
I retreat.

They beat attack,
but I dance just
out of reach—
lucky reaction time.

I parry riposte,
but it touches their arm.
Yellow light goes off:
touch off-target.

Fence!

They advance lunge.
Touch left.
That's bout.
5-0

THE LOVING LIFE SONNET

an amazing opportunity,
a chance i will never forget.
i wonder how everything came to be:
fun and happiness i will not regret.

light times of wonder,
dark times of despair:
some great fixings of things can occur,
but some things are broken beyond repair.

love pushes me forward, but fear pulls me back:
a battle to test my strength.
i hope it is not courage i will lack,
and i hope to go forward in great length.

i want to go out, yes, go out and dream.
i want to let my heart take me to where i will beam.

WINNER

Does anyone win?
Or maybe everybody wins?
Do only some people win?

Does everyone lose?
Do winners all have big trophies
or huge mansions?

Are winners the
people who find the joy
to live their lives to the fullest?

Do they cross the finish line first,
win the lottery,
or wear the prettiest clothes?

FALLEN FANTASIES

jubilant happiness
illuminated thoughts
fantasies
world-traveling
great adventure
happily-ever-after

no
metamorphic beginning
wretched tears
crumbled dreams
agony
problem
sadness-shrouded
no escape
no happily-ever-after

ROBOT

What's that
weird thing
on your arm?

Oh,
it's a continuous glucose monitor
that reads approximate blood glucose values
from my interstitial fluid
and then sends them to my basal rate modulator
    insulin pump.

Blank stare.

It helps me because my pancreas
doesn't work as well
as it should.

Well,
it makes you look
like a robot.

☙

It just helps me
with my Type 1 diabetes.

Eeew!
You have
diabetes?

Yes,
it's just an autoimmune …

Does that mean you
ate too much
sugar?

I look away.

☙

HOPE FOR THE CURE

Why does hope flow through my veins
while I coax the cure?
Despite sporadic gains,
why do I seek that evasive detour?

Doesn't exploring feel exciting and powerful—
passionately trying to make the future simpler?
Is working toward my ultimate goal
the ultimate form of pleasure?

I have worked so hard for over thirteen years
for modified stem cells under a microscope!
When the cure arrives, the world will cheer—
all because of a little something called hope.

WANTING A CURE
FOR TYPE 1 DIABETES

like getting second place
when i worked so hard to get first

like arriving on time at the airport
and realizing the flight is delayed

like climbing a mountain
and turning around because there is a storm at the top

like watching a chef
prepare my favorite food

like watching a storm and seeing the sun simultane-
ously,
knowing there will be a rainbow

but not yet

DREAM CATCHER

holding the great past
always there for reflection
showing dreams come true

DREAM

my innermost desire
wondering if it will ever come true
it comes to me at night
or in the day sometimes
in between
reality and fantasy

RESEARCH PAPER

"I know I am a freshman
not a scientist,
but can you find a paper about CRISPR in
Type 1 diabetes research?"

"Yes. Here's a paper."

"Thank you."

I can hardly stop myself from jumping up and down.

When I get home,
I take out the paper.
It is thick, and the title is
three lines long, and I
don't understand
most of the words.

Why am I doing this?
I ask myself after an
hour of reading
the first sentence to
decipher it.
It is like reading
in a different language.

When I see one word
I don't understand,
I look it up,
and the definition
has words I don't understand.
The cycle keeps going.

So, why am I doing this?
Because I want to help

find the cure for
Type 1 diabetes.
I am passionate
about making a difference
in Type 1 diabetes history.

BRAIN DISSECTION

Hippocampus.
Amygdala.
Yeah, I know about the brain.

I dissect it,
but I'm not afraid.
I don't get queasy,
or at least not that easy.

After the dissection,
we start brain trivia,
and I'm eager to prove I'm smart.

They call out the first question.
I don't understand.
Are they speaking English?
I have no idea.

I write down "frontal cortex"
just because my brain is all blank.

Did my brain disappear?
Or is it asleep?
What happened?

I look to see if anyone got the answer right
on this impossible question,
but everyone else did.
Is this a nightmare?

There was even a little girl
who got the answer right.
She looks like she's eight,
and she still skips, too.
She was grinning with her score of
500 points.

I had a grand
0 points.
Oh, great.

I tell myself,
that was only the first question—there are
plenty more chances.

But on the next question,
it's the same thing.
What are they saying?

and again and again
and again and again.

༄

LIFE

a great opportunity—
the greatest i will ever receive

made up of my experiences,
times essential to growth;
i grow in times of happiness,
while thankfulness, thoughtfulness, and knowledge
grow in times of sadness

i can contribute
to the world
just as one seed
can blow in the wind
and blossom into
giant trees
with strong roots

A Pair of Worn Shoes

a souvenir from a
long journey

showing how far
i have dared to venture

the question to ask is:
how will mine look?

Finger Stick

"Come on!
Let's check your
blood sugar."

"I'm scared.
Does it hurt?"

"No, I used to
prick my finger
every other hour."

My mom puts a
test strip in the meter.
She twists the checker,
loading it.

He gives my mom
his finger,
looking away.

"Are you ready?"
my mom asks.

꙳

"No!"
He pulls his finger
away.

She grabs his
finger now.
"Okay. 1…2…hey!"

He managed to
wriggle his finger
free from her tight grasp.

I did this when I was
one year old
about 12 times a day.
Why is it so hard?
It's just a drop of blood.

THE MOMENT IT CHANGED

I sat there—
completely stunned.
I always knew this would come,
but not at this moment—when it all changed.
This is the day when I am no longer a victim—
a victim of Type 1 diabetes.

We are strong.
We are powerful.
We are influential.
We are courageous.
We are the ones who
helped cure Type 1 diabetes.

This is what the day Type 1 diabetes is cured will look like.

#1: I AM

I am brave and cheerful.
I wonder why some people get Type 1 diabetes.
I hear everyone laughing.
I see a Hawaiian sunset at the beach.
I want to live a happy life.
I am brave and cheerful.

I pretend that happiness can solve everything.
I feel thankful that my family is happy and healthy.
I touch a beautiful flower.
I worry that I won't live a full life.
I cry because I laugh so much.
I am brave and cheerful.

I understand that I am lucky to be alive.
I say that hard work can help you accomplish anything.
I dream that one day I will make a difference in the world.
I try to always do my best at everything I do.
I hope that I will inspire others.
I am brave and cheerful.

TELL ME MORE

a mystery,
a story to be learned,
endless science;
words meant
to be said
by everyone;
the wonders of wondering

SNOWFLAKE

Intricately crafted,
a world of white
makes the long journey
from the sky.

From each,
a unique story
can be taught.

From each,
a unique story
can be learned.

THE ROSE WITH A THORN

Once upon a time,
in a beautiful garden near a splendid castle,
there was something extraordinarily beautiful.
It was a marvel for all to see.
It was blood-red, and the petals were unwrinkled and
    perfect.
It was, by far, the prettiest flower and rose in the garden.

But,
this magnificent rose had a thorn.
This thorn would prick the finger of anyone who
    attempted to pick it.
These unfortunate people had done no wrong:
they had simply appreciated the rose's beauty
and wanted to share that beauty with others.

Then one day,
a small girl from a faraway land came to the garden.
The girl gazed at the beautiful flowers,
but one flower caught her eye.
In all her life, she had never seen a more beautiful rose.

Upon seeing the rose,
she wanted to give it to her father as a gift
since he had done so much for her.

She approached the blood-red rose,
went up on her tiptoes,
and she stretched out her arm.
She tried to snap the rose's stem with her fingers,
but the rose stuck out its thorn.
The girl did not see the thorn and flicked her hand
    across it.

She came back to her father with no rose:
she came back to her father with blood caking
    her hand.
He expected his small girl to cry,
but not a tear was on her face.

She said to her father,
"Why, father, that rose has not yet learned to love.
It is beautiful, but it wants no goodness to be spread.
The rose uses its beauty wrongly, hurting others—
the beautiful rose with a thorn."

WORLD

a place of safety,
a place where
differences
are appreciated

a place of life,
a place where
every day is
a party

a place of happiness,
a place where
joy blooms
like flowers
in spring

a place of dreams,
a place where
"can't" does not
exist

a place of memories,
a place where
kindness and fun
are remembered

a place of beauty,
a place where
everyone's allure is
on the inside

a place of teamwork,
a place where
everyone has friends

a place of love,
a place where
the only type
of love is
unconditional love
for everything and everyone

⁓

Rock

all equal
no rock is best

all elegant and peaceful beings of nature
cherish simplicity

can we too be like rocks,
remaining unprejudiced,
non-judgmental,
open to the
wonderful world around us?

RIDE

galloping through the wilderness,
united as one,
walking,
trotting,
cantering,
galloping,
jumping,
leaping
for love,
for friendship,
for dreams
into the sunset,
silhouettes against the night sky

THE OCEANOGRAPHER, THE ASTRONOMER, AND THE GEOLOGIST

Three travelers embarked on a journey together.
One studied the ocean.
One studied the sky.
One studied the earth.

But one day,
as they were journeying,
the travelers started to argue.
Each individual believed their area of expertise to be
superior to the others.

The oceanographer answered,
"Oh, the vibrancy of life under the sea!
It is filled with wonders of the world,
if only one can appreciate it.

I dedicated my life to studying
these creatures, so fantastical
that one may think they are from another galaxy,
yet they are here on this very planet.

The water heals all pain—
both physically and mentally.
All pressure placed upon
one's shoulders is diminished,
and one becomes free.

When one is exploring the great sea,
they are free to sail wherever they choose.
If only they adjust their sails
to where they wish to venture."

The astronomer whispered,
"Think of the place above us:
where dreams are found and
come true.

Picture the night sky
and the telescope
with which you can see
everything you could ever dream of.

❧

Reach the sky, and there are
no limits as to what you can achieve,
if you believe in your
plane and your ability to steer it.

Imagine the place where you can
truly soar above all
and find liberty amidst the clouds."

The geologist asked,
"Yes, I agree,
but what about simply appreciating
where we were meant to be?

Where is a place that we humans
can adore more than this place
of life and journeys
which we call 'home'?

Why do we humans always yearn
for what we do not have,
even when this planet is all
we can ever dream of and more?

Who is incapable of loving
the place where the sky kisses the ocean,
the very place where we can plant seeds and help
    them grow,
where we can ground ourselves and make deep roots?"

Just then,
the three travelers happened upon
a beautiful sunset above the beach—
or maybe it was the sunrise.

IMAGINE

I am on top of the world.
The birds look like bugs,
the trees look like emeralds,
the houses look like doll houses,
the buildings look like lines, and
the airplanes look like eagles.

But,
I am sitting on the ground.
I look up to see the birds,
the trees,
the houses,
the buildings, and
the airplanes.

Imagine

#2: I AM

I am persevering, joyful, and compassionate.
I wonder what I will select to pursue in my life.
I hear angelic voices singing in impeccable harmony.
I see a magnificent Hawaiian sunset at the beach.
I want to spread my wings and soar in life.
I am persevering, joyful, and compassionate.

I pretend all my dreams will come true.
I feel love shrouding me.
I touch a shooting star.
I worry about the future of the world.
I cry when a valuable life has ceased to continue.
I am persevering, joyful, and compassionate.

I understand the world is not reliably just.
I say that all should feel as if their dreams are unlimited.
I dream that the world will change for the better.
I try to induce this difference in the world.
I hope everyone's wishes will come true.
I am persevering, joyful, and compassionate.

OPENNESS

free of judgement
without hate of any
religions,
genders,
races,
cultures

seeing differences
and admiring them

not looking down upon others,
but looking to everyone as equals

to embrace the unknown,
opening my eyes will do nothing,
so i open my heart

SUNSETS

a blend of colors
a methodical pattern
life is beautiful

RAIN

Swishh, Swshh
God is watering the
Earth to make
people happy.
Swshh, swshh!
Rain.

DONE

like circling my final answer
to a math problem

like playing the last
note of my violin piece

like sitting down after running
many miles

like slipping into
bed and closing my eyes

like reading the last sentence
of a book.

ACKNOWLEDGMENTS

Thank you to my amazing family! Mom, thank you for supporting me in everything I do and for asking me every day, "Have I told you yet today that I love you?" Dad, I love learning from your incredible perseverance and trying new and crazy things with you. Kelly, you will do great things with your infinite energy and beautifully powerful voice that lift me up. Kai, I know that I am older than you, but the best compliment I ever got was when someone said I was like you.

To my ohana, I love laughing and spending time with you! To my Grandma Brody, Grandma Gigi, Grandpa Dick, Papa, and Grandpa Arie in heaven, I will always remember to "Write with Eversharp," give arm kisses, savor life, love the ocean, and love my middle name.

To my friends, I can't frown because of you!

Thank you to the JDRF for giving me the best day of my life, the Hope Gala on my birthday. Thank you to Beyond Type 1 and diaTribe for educating our global community about diabetes. Also, thank you to diaTribe for such an incredible first job. Thank you to DYF for Bearskin Meadows and my first sleepaway camp.

Thank you to Eugene and Chee-Yun for teaching me to play beautiful music on my journey.

Thank you to the Oneder team of Jim, Linda, and Nancy for helping me make my dream of *Onederland* a reality.

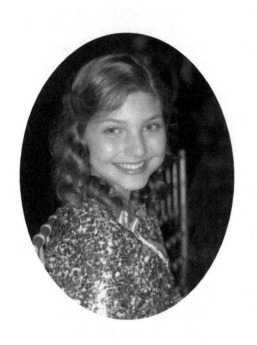

AUTHOR BIO

Jamie Kurtzig has been living with Type 1 diabetes since she was one year old, and she has been fighting for a cure ever since. As a child, she and her family created the Royal Ball, an annual family-friendly gala that raised over $1 million. In 2016, she began organizing the JDRF One Walk teams to raise money for Type 1 diabetes research, and she has raised over $55,000 with her walk team efforts so far. In 2018, Jamie was the Fund-A-Cure speaker at the JDRF Hope Gala in San Francisco and received the "Living and Giving" award. She and her family were the Honorees at this special event that raised over $2.8 million, and it was the happiest day of her life. Jamie is also a JDRF 2019 Children's Congress Delegate, a JDRF blogger (Looping with Jamie, Diary of an Artificial Pancreas, and Global T1D with Jamie: jdrf.org/kurtzigs), a JDRF Youth Ambassador at TypeOneNation Summits, a Junior Summer Associate at The diaTribe Foundation, and a volunteer working with continuous glucose monitors at Stanford University.

Jamie attends Marin Academy and Stanford Online High School. In her free time, she enjoys playing the violin, hanging out with her friends and family, traveling, fencing, and trying new and crazy things. Her goals are to publish a book, visit all seven continents, read Harry Potter in Spanish, play Piazzolla's "Porteña" on the violin, and make Type 1 diabetes history as a scientist by finding a cure.

✎

INDEX

Age 5
Rain 122

Age 7
Flying 76
Glasses 44
Imagine 118
Seasons 82
Wind to Earth 66

Age 9
A Feeling 78

Age 10
#1: I Am 105
Book 42
Butterfly's Wingbeat 48
Courage 13
Happiness 74
Pi 24
Poems 47
Sadness 34
Tell Me More 106

Age 11
Haiku 75

Age 12
#2: I Am 119

Beauty 41
Broken 29
Dream 95
Dream Catcher 94
Fallen Fantasies 89
Flower 79
Free Verse 22
Life 100
Lunar New Year 73
Maybe 64
Openness 120
Sunsets 121
The Loving Life Sonnet 87
The Taste of Victory 85
Trashcan 35
Water 23
World 110

Age 13
A Pair of Worn Shoes 101
Blue 55
Chocolate 54
Clock 12
Doctor 10
Hope for the Cure 92
Imagination 46
Jump 84
Name 10
Organization 20

Pen 45
Pen Pals a World Apart 57
Ride 113
Rock 112
Silence 36
Snowflake 107
Student 10
Taekwondo 21
The Moment It Changed 104
The Oceanographer,
   the Astronomer,
   and the Geologist 114
The Rose with a Thorn 108
Wanting a Cure for Type 1 Diabetes 93
Winner 88

Age 14
Aloha's Symphony 68
Audition 16
Bad Grade 65
Birthday Presents 58
Black Sand Beach 67
Brain Dissection 98
Can't 8
Celiac Disease 9
Cold 39
Cracking Knuckles 26
Done 123
Energy 50

Eyelashes 71
Family 37
Fashion 40
Fencing 86
Finger Stick 102
First Day of High School 38
Floating Wish Lantern 72
Gold 52
High Blood Sugar 11
How Long Is a Moment? 19
Low Blood Sugar 32
Moon 77
Music 18
¿Por Qué? / Why? (English Translation) 60, 61
Procrastination 28
Quartet 14
Rainy Day 43
Research Paper 96
Robot 90
Shooting Star 70
Sniffer 56
Sparring Tournament 4
Stress 30
Summer 83
Summer Day 49
Surprise 51
Think 25
Ukraine 62
Where I'm From 2
Wishing for Type 1 Diabetes 80

❧